PERSONAL GROWTH:
BOOK 1-3

Personal Growth: Book 1-3

BY LEE STRONG

TABLE OF CONTENTS

Mindfulness Meditation

Introduction..9

Chapter 1: Meditation..10

Chapter 2: How to Prepare Your Body and Mind for Meditation...14

Chapter 3: Best Music for Meditation..................................17

Chapter 4: Breathing Practices...20

Chapter 5: Sitting and Walking Meditation...........................23

Chapter 6: Practices of Senses...27

Chapter 7: Body Scan...32

Chapter 8: Meditation to Cope with Grief.............................37

Chapter 9: Informal Meditation Practice..............................39

Conclusion...42

Homo Arcticus Method: Book 1

Introduction...47

Chapter 1: Breathing..52

Chapter 2: Cold Therapy..57

Chapter 3: Commitment..64

Chapter 4: People's Experiences...69

Conclusion...71

Homo Arcticus Method: Book 2

Introduction – Who is Homo Arcticus?....................................75

Chapter 1: Homo Arcticus Discovery......................................77

Chapter 2: Homo Arcticus Method..79

Chapter 3: The Three Pillars...84

Chapter 4: Invest 2% of Energy to Achieve 100% Effectiveness...90

Chapter 5: Benefits of Homo Arcticus Method.........................92

Chapter 6: People's Experiences..95

Conclusion...96

Mindfulness Meditation

Guided Mindfulness Meditation for Beginners: Mindfulness Meditation Benefits, Breathing Techniques for Stress Relief, Music for Relaxation, Stress Relief, and Better Sleep

Introduction

This beginner's meditation book will help busy individuals to release tension, relieve stress, and reconnect with peace and tranquility. Today, millions of people around the world have taken up a meditation practice as a part of their everyday lives and with the help of this book, so can you! This meditation guidebook for beginners is a clear program for learning simple, but effective meditation techniques. Both newcomers and experienced meditators will enjoy the ease and variety presented in this book. This meditation book provides a range of meditation practices, with step-by-step guidance, and friendly advice so even a novice can practice.

Whether you like to practice in your home, at the office, on your commute, between appointments, or before sleep, this meditation book offers quick and easy guidance for instant wisdom, clarity, and calm. This beginner's guide offers you peace, clarity, and wisdom with just a few minutes of restful breathing a day. After reading this book, you will come away with a solid basis for your own meditation practice and for bringing meditation's remarkable benefits to every aspect of your life. Accessible and effective, this beginner's meditation book is a true how-to guide that will empower you to meditate with confidence right away.

Chapter 1: Meditation

The word "meditation" in Tibetan comes from the world "gom", which means, "to become familiar with." Meditation is a process of becoming familiar with life. You can do this by training your mind to pay attention. Most of the time we pay attention to our breath. Sometimes, we pay attention to a sound, a mantra, or what we are doing, such as walking, eating or showering. When we are completely focused on what is happening in the present, even for a few seconds at a time, we are not caught in the web of thoughts that constantly jumping between the future and the past. We become intimate with the experience of life and are able to live it more deeply.

Meditation is also the practice of coming home to ourselves. Even if for a single moment, you are not doing anything and you are just at your center, utterly relaxed - that is meditation. The time spent practicing being present with our breath trains out attention to be present more of the time in "regular" life off the meditation cushion. We start to notice as things arise and fall – in our emotions, in our bodies, and in nature. We listen when people talk to us rather than collecting the "gist" and then tuning out. We start to taste the food we eat, rather than mindlessly shoveling it in. Even as the chatter of our minds comes and goes, we stay rooted in life as it is happening, rather than got lost in repetitive thinking. We put down our busyness, distractions, our ideas about ourselves, and turn toward our lives.

The goal of the meditation practice is to make our mind calmer and peaceful. Daily meditation practice familiar our mind with virtue. Once we are acquainted with virtue, we will be calmer and peaceful. A *calm* and *peaceful* mind is *free* from mental discomfort, and worry, and it can then enjoy true happiness and bliss. Alternatively, if our mind is not calm and peaceful, we will find it challenging to enjoy true happiness even if we are living in comfort and have no reason to worry.

We could say that in essence, meditation is a direct and very convenient way to cultivate greater intimacy with your own life unfolding and with your inner capacity to be aware – and to realize how valuable, overlooked, and underappreciated an asset that awareness actually is.

The benefits of meditation

Here are the benefits of the meditation:

- Reduces stress: Most people practice meditation to lower stress. When you are stressed, cortisol, the stress hormone production increases. Studies show that excessive cortisol production can trigger inflammation. Inflammation can increase blood pressure, contribute to fatigue, disrupt sleep, promote anxiety and depression and results in cloudy thinking. Additionally, meditation can improve symptoms related to stress, including fibromyalgia, bowel syndrome, and post-traumatic stress disorder.
  [https://www.ncbi.nlm.nih.gov/pubmed/24395196
  http://www.sciencedirect.com/science/article/pii/S0889159112004758]

- Controls anxiety: Studies show meditation practice reduces anxiety and symptoms of anxiety disorders such as paranoid thoughts, social anxiety, phobias, panic attacks, and obsessive-compulsive behaviors.
  [http://www.sciencedirect.com/science/article/pii/016383439500025M
  https://onlinelibrary.wiley.com/doi/10.1002/da.21964/abstract]

- Promotes emotional health: Meditation practice can lead to a more positive outlook on life and an improved self-image. Various studies show meditation can lower depression. Also, meditation reduces inflammatory markers and lowers depression.

[http://www.sciencedirect.com/science/article/pii/016383439500025M
https://www.ncbi.nlm.nih.gov/pubmed/24439650]

- Boost self-awareness: The practice can transform you into a stronger individual. It can guide you to know yourself better and reach your fullest potential. Also, the practice can help cultivate more creative problem-solving.

  [https://www.ncbi.nlm.nih.gov/pubmed/26231761
  https://www.ncbi.nlm.nih.gov/pubmed/26686556]

- Improves your ability to focus: Daily meditation practice can help increase the strength and endurance of your attention. Various studies show that meditation practitioners can stay focused on a task for longer. A separate study even shows that meditation can prevent worrying, poor attention, and mind wandering.

  [https://link.springer.com/article/10.3758/CABN.7.2.109#page-1
  https://www.ncbi.nlm.nih.gov/pubmed/23643368]

- Can prevent memory loss: Meditation practice keeps your mind young and prevents age-related memory loss. Additionally, other studies show meditation can improve the memory of dementia patients.

  [https://www.ncbi.nlm.nih.gov/pubmed/26445019
  https://www.ncbi.nlm.nih.gov/pubmed/24571182]

- Fight addictions: Meditation practice increases your self-control and awareness and helps fight dependencies and addictions. Studies show that meditation increase willpower of the practitioners; boost their mental strength so they can control their emotions and stop addictive behaviors.

  [https://www.ncbi.nlm.nih.gov/pubmed/27012254

https://www.ncbi.nlm.nih.gov/pubmed/26784917]

- Improves sleep: Insomnia is a big problem for most people. The study shows that meditation practice helps practitioners get better quality sleep when compared with people who do not meditate. Also, the practice can release bodily tension, relax your body and place you in a peaceful state. All three promotes better sleep.

[https://www.ncbi.nlm.nih.gov/pubmed/26390335]

- Help control pain: Your mind controls your perception of pain and if you are stressed, then your pain can increase. The study shows that meditation practitioners feel less sensitivity to pain. Another study shows that meditation can lower chronic pain.

[https://www.ncbi.nlm.nih.gov/pmc/articles/PMC3090218/

https://www.ncbi.nlm.nih.gov/pubmed/24395196]

- Lower blood pressure: The practice reduces strain on the heart by lowering blood pressure. High blood pressure can lead to heart attacks and strokes.

[https://www.ncbi.nlm.nih.gov/pubmed/25673114

https://www.ncbi.nlm.nih.gov/pubmed/25390009]

Chapter 2: How to Prepare Your Body and Mind for Meditation

Here are tips on how to prepare yourself for meditation practice:

1. Initiate your motivation. Know why you want to meditate. Perhaps you want to relieve stress or improve your focus, or you may want to sleep better or want to achieve inner peace. Don't judge your reasons as being good or bad. Just recognize them as they are. Knowing your reasons for motivation will help you deal with any feelings of resistance or restlessness and help you focus.

2. Set realistic goals. Set goals that you can achieve. This way, you will not get disappointed. As a beginner, you should choose simple goals such as practicing daily for 20 minutes and not giving up and so on.

3. Beware of expectations. Don't expect to become a meditation expert within days after practice. Even experienced meditation practitioners reveal that they also occasionally get distracted or lose focus when practicing. Instead of trying to get everything perfect, focus on mimicking exercises as accurately as possible. Don't think that I can't do it or I can't get it right.

4. Prepare your environment. Ideally, you should practice in a quiet space. It could be your home or in your office. If you are practicing in your home, then the morning time is the best time to practice. It is usually peaceful in the morning and easier to create an environment that will enhance your

practice. If you are practicing in your office then hang a "please do not disturb" sign on your door or choose a spot with fewer distractions. Playing gentle music while your meditation is a good idea. Soothing and relaxing music can actually help you focus.

5. Don't eat a heavy meal before practice. If you must eat, then eat a snack before practice. Eating a heavy meal might make it difficult to sit comfortably for the practice. Also, a meal before practice can make you feel sleepy.

6. Deal with distraction: Complete silence is rare. So learn to deal with the distraction. Kids are playing in the distance, or cars driving by or even a dripping faucet can distract a beginner. Try to lower distractions as much as possible. However, with time you will discover that some external noise is helping to develop your sense of hearing and observation.

7. It is not mandatory, but you can shower before practice. This act of cleansing yourself before practice has a symbolic significance. It can have a positive effect on you, especially if you are a beginner. Additionally, a hot bath before practice will make your body relax by wash away all the muscular tension.

8. Wear loose-fitting clothes that make you comfortable and help you focus. Make sure that the space in which you meditate is not too hot or too cold.

9. Do some stretches before practice to relax any tension in your body and muscles. Take a few minutes to stretch and breathe deeply. Especially focus on your head, neck and leg muscles. Stretching and taking deep breathes will relax your body, mind, and emotions.

10. Sit in a comfortable position. Here is a checklist for sitting:

Sit comfortably and keep your back, neck, and head aligned. Don't lean backward or forward. Keep your muscles balanced by keeping your hands level and shoulders even.

You can keep your eyes closed or opened, whichever makes you comfortable.

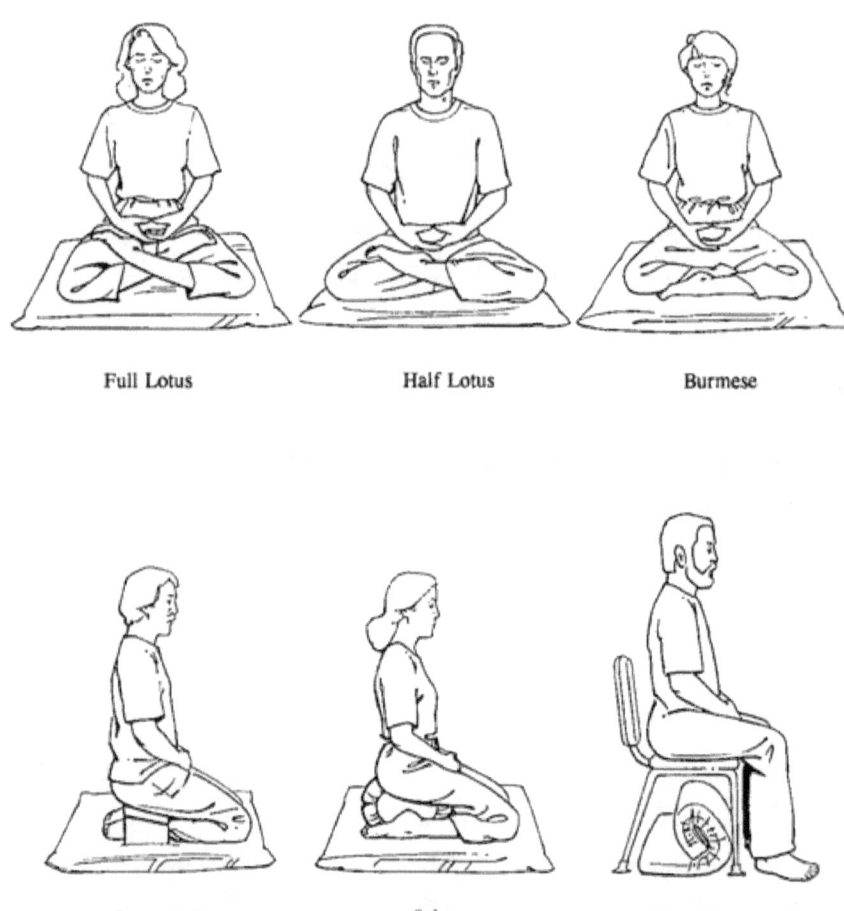

| Full Lotus | Half Lotus | Burmese |

| On a stool | Seiza | On a Chair |

Chapter 3: Best Music for Meditation

Here are some music choices that you might find helpful during practice:

1. Arvo Pärt: Spiegel im Spiegel

   https://www.youtube.com/watch?time_continue=82&v=z8ZScAdV8qE

2. Alexis Ffrench – Radiate

   https://www.youtube.com/watch?v=wlWsDwY8p2Y

3. Jan Sandström: Det är en ros utsprungen

   https://www.youtube.com/watch?v=86-ulHbApOM

4. Max Richter: Dream 3

   https://www.youtube.com/watch?v=AwpWZVG5SsQ

5. Debussy: Clair de Lune

   https://www.youtube.com/watch?v=LlvUepMa31o

6. John Tavener: The Last Sleep of the Virgin

   https://www.youtube.com/watch?v=M-RyBCFc76k

7. Morten Lauridsen: O Magnum Mysterium

   https://www.youtube.com/watch?list=RDOj9-2RgM6p4&v=Q7ch7uottHU

8. Erik Satie: Gnossiennes

   https://www.youtube.com/watch?v=5pyhBJzuixM

9. Thomas Newman: Any Other Name

   https://www.youtube.com/watch?v=kY7eYJOasuI

10. Charles Villiers Stanford: The Bluebird

    https://www.youtube.com/watch?v=nE0JRx3CHv8

11. Erik Satie: Gymnopedie No.1

    https://www.youtube.com/watch?v=WcfxFxWI9R8

12. Eric Whitacre: Lux Aurumque

    https://www.youtube.com/watch?v=0j2JRcC6wBs

13. Philip Glass: Satyagraha, 'Evening Song'

    https://www.youtube.com/watch?v=qBIw017cq4k

14. The Best Relaxing Classical Music Ever By Chopin

    https://www.youtube.com/watch?v=Iz07rd3qsSs

15. Classical Chillout - Pachelbel, Mozart, Beethoven, Debussy, Janacek, Bach, Handel

    https://www.youtube.com/watch?v=hSnD30bcAS8

16. The Best Of YIRUMA Yiruma's Greatest Hits

    https://www.youtube.com/watch?v=9L5cdoBPryY

17. Relaxing Music for Stress Relief. Calm Celtic Music for Meditation, Healing Therapy, Sleep, Yoga

    https://www.youtube.com/watch?v=6xDyPcJrl0c

18. Relaxing Music for Meditation. Calm Background Music for Stress Relief, Sleep, Yoga, Massage, Spa

    https://www.youtube.com/watch?v=sDuadJovyBE

19. The Best Relaxing Classical Music Ever By Beethoven - Relaxation Meditation Focus Reading

    https://www.youtube.com/watch?v=_rS8N7-tnzw

20. 8 HOURS Relaxing Music for Stress Relief {Completely Beat Insomnia} Music for Deep Sleep, Meditation

    https://www.youtube.com/watch?v=mFlrc16xjik

Here are other collections:

1. *https://itunes.apple.com/us/album/50-best-meditation-songs-collection/1110324990*

2. *https://open.spotify.com/album/67ozVdV9kfSsWizbxWEIcc*

3. *https://soundcloud.com/meditation-music*

Chapter 4: Breathing Practices

In this chapter, we are going to discuss breathing exercises that are an integral part of meditation practice.

Steps to initiate diaphragmatic breathing:

1. Assume a comfortable position. You can practice this exercise anywhere, at any time. To start, get into a comfortable position, either sitting or, lying down on your back. Place your hands over your stomach and feel the rise and fall of your abdomen with each breath. When you master the technique, you can do it anywhere, even when driving in heavy traffic, or waiting in line at the post office.

2. Concentration: Diaphragmatic breathing requires focused concentration. Limit distraction to enhance your ability to concentrate. Concentration can be augmented further by focusing on the components of each breath. Each ventilation is said to be composed of four distinct phases:

    Phase one: Inspiration, or taking the air into your lungs through the nose or mouth

    Phase two: A very slight pause before exhaling

    Phase three: Exhalation, or releasing the air from your lungs through the passage it entered

    Phase four: Another very slight pause after exhalation before the next inhalation is initiated

The practice:

1. You can practice this exercise standing, sitting or lying on your back. You can close your eyes or keep them open.

2. Take a moment to loosen your body, especially your jaws, upper chest, and shoulders. Bring your awareness to each of these parts of the body. Then relax any tenseness you find there. Imagine your breath softening any tight areas.

3. Bring your awareness to your breath. Focus as your breath enters through your nose and exists through your mouth.

4. Breathe in for 3 seconds and out for 3 seconds.

5. Rest one hand on your belly and the other hand on your chest.

6. As you inhale, allow your stomach and waist expand outward.

7. Your hand on your chest should hardly move at all. In contrast, your abdomen should move downward as it contracts.

8. This completes one round. Now repeat steps 4 to 7 a few times.

When you have finished practicing, relax both arms and breathe naturally for a few moments.

Deconstructed Breath

This mindfulness practice encourages you to explore the upper, middle and lower regions of the torso through your breath. The aim is to breathe sequentially into each area. First, fill the lower torso, then fill the rib cage and chest area.

The practice:

1. Sit in a comfortable pose. Keep your eyes closed or open.

2. Soften your body, especially your jaws, upper chest, and shoulders. Bring your awareness to each of these body parts one by one. Then loose, and relax any tenseness or tightness you notice.

3. Start to breathe in and out through your nose.

4. As you breathe in, draw about one-third of the breath into your lower belly. Let your stomach and waist to expand outward. Then draw another one-third of the breath into your rib cage and let the ribs to expand to the back, sides, and front of your torso. Draw the last one-third of your breath into your upper chest. Let your breastbone rise slightly.

5. When exhaling, release one-third of the breath from your upper chest. Observe that your breastbone sink slightly. Then release one-third of the breath from the rib cage and let the rib cage sink in the middle of your body. Release the final one-third of your exhalation from your lower belly.

6. This finishes one round. Repeat steps 4 to 5 a few times.

7. When finished, simply stay still and breathe normally for a few seconds.

Chapter 5: Sitting and Walking Meditation

In this chapter, we are going to discuss sitting and walking meditation.

Sitting meditation

The practice:

- Sit comfortably and close your eyes.

- Begin by gently moving your attention to the process of breathing. Take three gentle, deep breaths. Then start to breathe naturally. Allow the breath to breathe itself.

- Let go of any effort to focus, and simply leave your mind alone. You will soon notice that your mind starts to chatter. It might start to show you tempting and pleasurable things – such as the sports match you are going to view this evening or the delicious dinner you are going to cook tomorrow. Just like an untrained puppy, your mind might begin to run toward these tantalizing things, but try not to chase them. Don't try to forcefully get rid of your pleasurable thoughts. Just let them be and avoid getting caught up in chasing them. Let them go.

- Your mind might also present you with stressors, problems, and worries such as your job situation, work conflicts, world politics, and so on. Let the unsettling thoughts be there with you. Don't worry about how long they are there. Don't try to remove them or push them away. Let them be, but let them go.

- If your thoughts are like clouds (and your mind is the sky) coming and taking center stage for a moment. Don't worry about unwanted activity finding your mind space. Just notice your thoughts without analyzing them or judging them. As you continue to allow thoughts to come and go, you will also begin to experience the spaces between them. You don't need to do anything in these empty spaces. Allow yourself to just sit, and be. Soon, other thoughts will arise. Notice it and let it go. If necessary, return to your breath to center yourself.

- When you are ready to end your practice, take a few moments to expand your awareness back to your breath and into the room around you. Become aware of the sounds and scents around you. Become aware of your body. When you feel ready, open your eyes.

Mindful Walking

Mindful walking is an ancient and effective practice for cultivating mindfulness. To practice, choose a spot where you can walk at least 12 steps before needing to turn. You can practice in your home or on beaches and fields. Remove your shoes and practice:

The practice:

1. Stand still and start to settle your awareness into your body and onto your breath. Acknowledge to yourself that you are about to start the practice of mindful walking.

2. Start walking. Move your body with intent, but try not to change the way you are walking – just observe yourself.

3. Bring all of your attention to the sensations within your body

4. Start with your feet. Notice which part of your foot leaves the ground first, and which part touches it first. Observe how your toes respond to the motion of walking.

5. Notice your knee and ankle joints. See how they flex, extend, and absorb impact.

6. Become aware of the muscles in your thighs. Notice how they contract and flex as you move.

7. Observe your hips and pelvis and how they move. Notice their multidirectional movements, and how they rotate and sway. Do these movements feel clunky or smooth to you?

8. Explore the movements and sensations within your upper body. Notice how your opposite shoulder and hip movement in alignment through the gentle twist of your torso.

9. Observe how your body feels as a whole. Does it feel heavy or light?

10. Shift your attention to your environment. Turn your awareness away from your body and toward the environment around you. Acknowledge what you see without analyzing it. Is your mind tempted to engage with the things you observe? If so, notice it and let it go.

Chapter 6: Practices of Senses

In this chapter, we are going to discuss the practices of senses.

The five senses

The five senses practice will help come to your senses, feel grounded and be in the present moment. It offers a gentle inroad into an alert, but a relaxed mental state, which is the foundational mind state of meditation. Through this practice, you will also begin practicing the fundamental attitudes of meditation by cultivating your capacity to bring freedom, spaciousness, and curiosity.

The practice:

- Sit comfortably.

- Take three deep breaths, then start to breathe normally. Don't try to slow it down or speed it up. Just breathe normally.

- Now try to listen to everything you hear. Focus on the sounds around you. Notice the most prominent sound first. Then one by one notice all the quitter sounds all around you. Even try to notice the faintest sound you can hear. There might be sounds that are generating within your body.

- Then, focus your attention to everything you can smell. Stay non-judgmental and objective. Just like before, notice the most noticeable smell you can detect. If you can't detect any smell, then it is okay, too. Remember, an absence of smell is also an experience. Try to smell all the things you can smell. It might be the fragrance of flowers or the fragrance of food. Don't try to label the smells as "good" or "bad". Just notice them as they are without labeling them.

- Now, focus your attention to everything you can taste. Try to taste without judgment or observation. You may still taste the coffee you just drink. Or the chewing gum you chew a few minutes ago. If you can't taste anything then it is okay because the absence of taste is also an experience.

- Now, move your attention and focus to your sense of touch. Focus on your body and try to notice all the feeling you get on your skin. Maybe it is an ache or physical discomfort. Scan your whole body to find any sense of touch. Maybe you feel your stomach gurgling or your right foot might be about to fall asleep.

- Lastly, move your attention to your sense of vision. If you are sitting beside a window, then look at the sky to see the clouds or the absence of clouds. From your window, you might see your backyard or cars driving by. Notice the most prominent one then gradually go to the most obscure one. If you can't see anything then it is okay too.

Practice daily for 10 to 20 minutes and spend 2 to 4 minutes exploring each of your senses.

The six senses practice

The six senses practice builds upon the five senses practice. You will learn to use the traditional five senses as gateways to explore the present moment and then to enter into the spaciousness that exists when you allow all of these senses to be awake, alive, open, and aware at the same time.

The practice:

1. Sit comfortably.

2. Start by gently shifting your attention to the process of breathing. Take three, full, deep breaths. Notice the sound of your breath and the movement of your upper body. Then allow your breath to settle into a natural rhythm.

3. Bring your attention to everything you hear. Notice the sounds around you. First, notice the most prominent sound you can detect. Then one by one observe all of the quieter sounds in your surrounding environment. Even notice the sounds your body is making. Notice them, but don't judge them or analyze them.

4. Now shift your attention and focus on everything you can smell. If you can't smell anything, it is fine. Remember, no experience is also an experience. Explore your sense of smell, but without judgment. There is no such thing as "good" or "bad".

5. Move your attention and focus on everything you can taste. Perhaps your breath. Maybe you can taste the alkaline or acidic taste of your own saliva. Or maybe you can still taste the chewing gum you chew a few minutes ago. Simply notice without judging or analyzing.

6. Now, move your attention and focus on everything you can feel with your skin. Maybe the prickle of goosebumps, the warmth of sunlight, or the way the feeling of your shirt on your skin. Do so with a nonjudgmental openness and curiosity.

7. Now, keep your eyes closed and shift your attention and focus on everything you can see behind your eyelids. Be wide open to whatever your experience bursts or washes of color, pinpoints of light or sheer blackness.

8. Now turn your attention back toward your own mind, toward your sixth sense – the awareness of your own thinking. In your mind's eye, open the backs of your eyes, and your inner ears by imagining them. See how they, too, turn inward with intent and awareness. Observe mind stuff arising and passing away.

9. Notice your thoughts. Like a fast, powerful river, they may be rushing past, or they might be trickling, like a gentle stream. Maybe there is a still and silent backdrop behind them, or perhaps there is space between thoughts. Simply watch your own mind.

10. Now become aware of that you who are watching your mind. Become aware of awareness itself. Be aware of the sense of awareness from which you have observed your own mind. Curiously notice the undercurrent of awareness. Be conscious of your own presence.

11. Let your awareness encompass all your senses at once: sights, textures, tastes, smell, sounds, and the mind itself – awareness itself. Don't worry if that doesn't last for very long. It is completely normal to have a sense of the "whole" of these experiences, only to have that moment crumble. Simply

keep opening yourself to experiencing all of your senses at once, again and again.

12. Try to sense how the experiences of this world continue to play through you, without in any way limiting or capturing the inborn capaciousness of awareness. You are utterly awake, utterly open. You are the sky with the birds flying through it. You are the awareness itself. Notice this awareness.

13. At the end of the practice, take a few moments to expand your awareness from your breath into the room around you. Become aware of the scents and sounds around you. Become aware of your body. Gently wiggle your fingers and toes. When you feel ready, open your eyes.

Chapter 7: Body Scan

The body scan meditation

The body scan meditation gives you the unique opportunity to practice mindfulness lying down. This makes it a perfect meditation for beginners. You can practice body scan at any time of the day.

The exercise:

1. Rest into a comfortable position: Lie on your back, keep your legs a little apart from each other and arms a bit away from the sides of your body with your palms facing up. Your body temperature may drop when you practice, so cover yourself with a blanket if you need to. If this position is uncomfortable, then choose a position that feels right for you.

2. Focus on your inner attitude: Allow and accept whatever happens in the practice as best as you can, let it be. Let go of any notion of personal development or self-improvement. Mindfulness is all about allowing yourself to be as you are in a deep, authentic and meaningful way.

3. Breathe: For a few minutes, just focus your attention on your breathing.

4. Step by step, move your attention through your entire body: Move your focus from your breathing down to the toes, try to feel whatever sensation you can feel. If you can't feel any sensation in your toes, just be mindful of the absence of sensation. One after another, shift your focus to –

I. Your feet

II. Lower part of your legs

III. Upper part of your legs

IV. Pelvic region

V. Lower part of the torso

VI. Upper part of the torso

VII. Your shoulders

VIII. Hands

IX. Your Lower arms

X. Upper arms

XI. Your neck

XII. Back of your head

XIII. Face

XIV. Finish with the top of your head

It should take you about 15 to 30 minutes to finish the complete the practice. Mind wandering is common. So, don't get discouraged and bring your attention to your breathing every time you lose focus.

5. Imagine your breath covering your entire body: When you breathe in, imagine your breath starting from your toes and finishing at the top of your

head. When you breathe out, imagine your out-breath sweeps from the top of the head down to your toes. This bodily sensation should feel relaxing or healing.

6. For the last few minutes of your meditation, let go all your effort to be mindful and just allow things to happen. Rest in your own inner sense of presence, of aliveness, of being.

7. Gently stand up: Gradually bring the meditation to a close. Get up gradually and mindfully, avoid jumping up straight away because it may make you feel dizzy. Feel the sensation in your body.

Overcoming difficulty with the body scan

Following are a few problems you may experience during the practice of body scan.

- You falling asleep: Feeling sleepy or falling asleep is a normal occurrence during practice, but the idea of the meditation is to "become more aware of the surroundings and your feelings" rather than actually falling asleep. Change your practice time to avoid falling asleep, practice body scan and keep your eyes open instead of closing them or take a cool shower before the practice. If you still have a falling asleep problem, then practice meditation sitting in a chair, and keep your back relaxed and loose. The crucial thing is to keep practicing, even if you feel sleepy during practice.

- Unable to feel any bodily sensation: When practicing, if you can't feel or sense any bodily sensation in a specific or large part of the body, then it's okay, and don't worry about it. Just acknowledge the absence of sensation and accept it – this is the core of mindfulness. With practice, you will feel more bodily sensation.

- You feel stressed or more anxious: Occasionally you may not find the mindfulness practice of body scan soothing. After several sessions of practice, if you still find the practice not working, then you may be hoping to achieve a higher standard or trying too hard. Try to let go of that idea, don't be critical or harsh with yourself.

- You feel restless or bored: You are really busy and active individual, so you may find the body scan really boring and feel restless during practice. Utilize the boredom in a positive way; try to observe the feeling of restlessness or boredom within your body. Don't try to push these feelings away, and focus on the feelings of restlessness or boredom.

Chapter 8: Meditation to Cope with Grief

In this chapter, we are going to discuss meditation to deal with grief.

Grief

Grief can be exhausting. Meditation can provide our tired, grieving hearts and minds with respite. It can replenish our nervous system, and it can help us be present with ourselves. Remaining present with grief facilitates healing. Remember, however strong your grief may be, it is also entirely ordinary and it is an integral part of being human.

The practice:

1. Sit in any position that is comfortable for you, and close your eyes.

2. Begin by gently moving your attention to the process of breathing. Take three, full, deep breaths. Feel your abdomen as you inhale, and allow your entire body to soften as you exhale. Then start to take gentle breaths.

3. Rest your attention on the anchor of your breath or another anchor such as S sound or a mantra. Soon you will notice that your mind starts to get distractions with feelings, thoughts, and sensations.

4. When the feeling of grief arises, allow the feeling to take the center stage. Leave your anchor (your breathing or a mantra) knowing that you can come back to it at any moment. Allow your mind to wander to any aspect of your grief.

5. Label the aspects of grief that arise in your mind as "worrying," "anger", "remembering,", or "reminiscing" or whatever else comes up for you. All these manifestations are facets of your grief. Allow them to be present, and let them wash in and out of your awareness.

6. Now, notice the part of you that is watching these experiences within your own mind. Become aware of awareness itself, and ask yourself whether this aware part of you actually dwells in grief. Even though you are in the midst of the emotion, you will probably discover that the answer is no. This suggests that there are aspects of your being that are larger than your suffering and your grief. Awareness is *larger* than grief.

7. Allow your awareness to gently hold the space in which your grief is present. Cradle both yourself and the emotion in the loving embrace of your all-encompassing, compassionate awareness. Accept whatever arises. It is okay if you start to cry. Allow it to happen and keep on cradling yourself and this grief.

8. When you are ready to complete your practice, return your awareness to your breath and enjoy three full, conscious breaths. Become aware of the space around you before you slowly open your eyes.

Chapter 9: Informal Meditation Practice

Alongside formal practices of meditation, informal practices of meditation can be a much larger part of our lives than we can ever imagine.

Mindful Eating

Here is how you can make your eating as an effective practice of meditation:

The practice:

1. Sit down at the dining table, preferably alone. Focus on your breaths as it comes in and goes out of your body and relax.

2. Take your time and appreciate the food that is in front of you. The food that you are going to eat might have ingredients from different countries of the world. Appreciate the hard work that has gone into preparing your food, from crop cultivation to food preparation. More than anything, show gratitude that you actually have food in your place because there are people out there in the world starving at this moment. You are grateful that you are not one of them.

3. If you are going to eat your food by hand, then notice the temperature, texture, and color of the food as you pick it up and move it towards your mouth. If you are using a fork or a spoon, then notice the texture of the spoon or fork that you are holding. Spend enough time noticing your food before you start to eat it.

4. Notice the distinct aromas of your food, as it gets closer to your mouth. Make it a point to savor your food before it finally caresses your tongue. When your food touches your tongue for the first time, be aware of the taste and texture of the food before it makes its way down towards your digestive system.

5. As you start to chew your food, you will notice that your mind has started making comparisons with the various meals that you have eaten earlier, such as it is too hot or cold, spicy or has a sweet taste. Remain as passive as possible with your thoughts and chew your food completely. This will assist you to appreciate each and every single mouthful of food that you are eating.

6. After you have eaten a few mouthfuls of food, you will notice that your mind has started to wander off again. When it happens, just notice where your mind went and then return your focus on the tastes, textures, smell, and sight of your food that is in front of you. As you start to get full, you will feel a little discomfort. Make a note of this in your mind and continue to eat until your meal is finally finished.

Showering for Mindfulness

You can start your day with meditation practice by incorporating it with your early morning shower. Practicing meditation while you take a hot shower makes it more enjoyable.

The practice:

1. Make sure your smartphone and other distractions such as TV and radio are turned off. You don't want anyone or anything disturbing you while you take a shower, mindfully.

2. As soon as you step into the shower, try to be aware of all the little things that are a part of taking your shower. Begin by noticing the temperature of the shower handle and its texture as you turn on the shower.

3. Notice the sound of the shower water. Be aware of the difference between the sound of the shower while you are standing under it and when the water directly hits the floor.

4. Feel the sensation of the water on your body; notice how easily it glides over your skin. Feel other sensations like if the water is hot or cold. Notice all the smells and feelings that are associated with the shampoo, soap and even the shower itself.

5. Notice any disruptive thoughts that might try to enter your mind while you are focused on your shower. Make sure that you are truly enjoying your shower.

Conclusion

Through various scientific studies, meditation is recognized as a highly effective tool for dealing with stress, anxiety, lowering blood pressure and other mental and physical illness. Meditation isn't about chanting, looking at crystals, or playing with an eagle feather. It is a scientifically proven way of taking control of your *life* by taking control of your *mind*. Daily meditation practice can make you healthier, happier, and more successful than ever. Only a few minutes of meditation practice daily can help you lower stress, improve your mental and physical health, boost your focus and increase work productivity. If you heard about meditation but don't know how to begin – or you have practiced meditation in the past, but need help to get started again, this beginner's meditation guidebook is for you.

Accessible and portable, this beginner's meditation guidebook offers simple but powerful meditation techniques that positively impact every area of physical and mental health. Whether this is your first experience with meditation practice, or you have practiced before, this book will transform your relationship with yourself and the world around you. This book opens the door to a life lived in the freedom of your innermost being. We hope that this book is going to help you to find best method for mindfulness meditation, useful exercises and practices, good music suggestions for relaxation, stress relief and better sleep. We encourage you to try implementing meditation to your everyday life because we live in stressful time and our mental and physical health could depend on it.

Homo Arcticus Method: Book 1

How Power Breathing Technique, Extreme Cold Therapy and Strong Commitment Can Make You Strong, Healthy, Happy and Change Your Life Forever

Introduction

We live in a very unhealthy world today - junk foods, polluted environment, not so fresh air, zero or minimal exercise, and reduced sleeping times.

All of these contribute to the growth and spread of diseases in the world today. It always seems like a new type of disease or virus is discovered every day.

But let me take you back to a few thousand years ago when our ancestors lived in the wild without clothes, access to advanced medicine or even a roof over their heads. They survived, didn't they?

They trekked for thousands of miles to gather food and supplies yet they didn't drop dead on the way. Many of us in this generation cannot even ride a bicycle for 5 kilometers.

One of the reasons why our hunter-gatherer ancestors were able to survive in those extreme living and weather conditions is because they had stronger immune systems. Think of the immune system as the engine room of your entire body. Your immune system is a network of organs, proteins, tissues, and cells, which work together to defend your body, and provide resistance to toxins, bacteria, viruses, parasites and other foreign bodies that cause diseases and illnesses.

When your immune system is strong enough and working as it should, it becomes very difficult for bacteria and viruses that cause diseases to thrive within your body. Everything that poses a threat to your body is quickly identified and eliminated before it gets a chance to wreak havoc.

A healthy and strong immune system equals a strong and healthy body and our hunter-gatherer ancestors had this going for them.

They could pick fruits and nuts from the wild to eat without cooking (maybe they didn't even wash the fruits sometimes because the nearest stream would be kilometers away) yet there was no extinction-level cholera or virus that wiped the entire human race out.

They survived the harshest of conditions but some of us can't even go outside our homes without a sanitizer or we'll get very sick.

The truth is that as the human race became more civilized, our immune systems, physical abilities and survival skills became weaker.

We got too comfortable and became weaklings; sorry it's harsh but true.

It's unlikely that we can stop people from polluting the air so that we can breathe in fresher air.

Packaged foods filled with chemical preservatives do not seem to be going out of fashion anytime soon. And it doesn't look like employers are going to start giving us sleeping holidays.

All the factors that contribute to making us unhealthy and weak humans are still going to be there at least for the foreseeable future so how do you look out for yourself and protect yourself?

How do you make your body healthier, stronger and able to withstand tough conditions without breaking down?

The Homo Arcticus method provides the answers.

Who is Homo Arcticus?

He is a 58-year old Dutch extreme athlete and fitness guru who has been nicknamed *"Homo Arcticus"* thanks to his impressive ability to withstand extreme cold.

He is that guy who climbed to the tops of Mounts Everest and Kilimanjaro wearing a pair of shorts and shoes. Mount Everest is the highest mountain in the world, rising a staggering 29,029 feet and temperature levels that can go up to -32C or more.

More than 200 people have died trying to climb Mount Everest fully clothed, but here's this guy climbing this mountain almost naked and he makes it all the way up and down without incident- no mountain sickness.

He repeated the same feat at the Mount Kilimanjaro, the tallest mountain in Africa, which stands at 19, 340 feet and temperature levels that can go up to -15C on 'warm' days.

If you think those are the only feats that earned him this title, you're wrong.

He has performed more than 26 seemingly impossible feats and has the Guinness World Titles to show for it.

- He completed a full marathon above the Arctic Circle wearing a pair of black shorts and shoes.

- He ran a full Marathon in the Namibian Desert without water.

- He took an ice bath for almost 2 hours- and by that, I mean that he sat in a tub that was filled with ice up to his neck.

- He once hung on a finger at an altitude of 2,000 meters.

Of course, people started to question- how is this man able to do all of these?

He was quick to explain the logic behind his crazy endurance levels.

He explained that he mastered the ability to control his body temperatures, and literally turn up his own thermostat by using his mind. He is able to use his mind to send messages to his brain and all other parts of his body, telling them to keep warm even when external temperatures are crazy.

And before he was able to master this level of control over his mind and body, he has to learn three things which make up the pillars of the Homo Arcticus Method and anyone can replicate his results just by mastering these three pillars too.

The *Three Pillars* of the Homo Arcticus Method include:

- **Breathing**: Learning how to take control of your breathing can help you regain control of your entire body.

  Taking charge of how you breathe helps you intentionally reduce your stress levels, give you more energy, helps your muscles perform at optimal levels, and improve your immune system function by increasing oxygen consumption and metabolism.

  In short, learning how to breathe properly gives you control of your body's fight or flight response.

- **Cold Therapy**: Cold therapy involves exposing your body to cold temperatures and training your body to withstand extreme temperature without breaking down.

  Cold therapy causes your body to release more endorphins. Endorphins are the same chemicals that are released in your body when you work out or engage in serious physical activity and cold therapy makes your body release more of these chemicals as though you were working out.

  Endorphins interact with the pain receptors in your brain to reduce your ability to feel pain.

Endorphins also make feel good, prevent stress, and wards off feelings of anxiety and depression.

It helps to improve sleep quality, boost self-esteem, and make you feel good, really.

Cold therapy also plays a role in helping to improve your metabolism, reduce inflammation, regulate your hormone levels, and help you lose weight faster (fat loss).

- **Commitment**: The third pillar of the Homo Arcticus method is commitment. Yes, the Homo Arcticus method teaches you self-mastery.

  When you're able to control your mind and how it works and responds, you are also able to control every other aspect of your life; whether it's how you eat, your attitude towards work, your spending patterns, your relationships, and every other aspect of your life.

Read on to learn more about the Homo Arcticus method, and how to master the three pillars easily.

Thanks again for purchasing this book. We hope you enjoy it!

Chapter 1: Breathing

The Homo Arcticus breathing technique involves a repeated cycle of big inhalations followed by brief periods of holding your breath.

Basically, you have to take 30-40 power breaths, followed by holding your breath for increasingly long periods of time.

When you start out, you may not be able to hold your breath for too long but as you continue to train, you'll be able to improve on your breath retention.

The cool thing about this breathing exercise is that it can be done almost anywhere - while waiting in line for your coffee or sitting at your favorite restaurant - the only rule is that it has to be done without interruptions.

Caution: Please don't do this while driving especially if you're new to Homo Arcticus training.

It takes just a few minutes to do the exercise and doing it everyday increases your ability to control your breathing, and unlocks all of the benefits of Homo Arcticus breathing.

Recommendation for exercise: Homo Arcticus personally suggests doing the breathing exercise in a comfortable sitting or lying position and preferably in the morning on an empty stomach before breakfast. However, you can do it any way you prefer it to do. The most important thing is that you need to feel comfortable and focused on breathing (more than thinking or counting breath retention time).

Breathing Techniques and Exercises

Step One: Find a comfortable position. Look for a place that is comfortable-where you can sit or lie down for a few minutes without disturbance.

Step Two: Breathe in and out normally a few times - this is just prep for the main exercise.

Step Three: Now take 30-40 deep breaths at a steady pace (inhale and exhale continuously).

Don't inhale fully or too deeply - inhale until your belly rises halfway, and exhale until your belly falls back a bit but not completely.

It's going to look like you're hyperventilating when you do it repeatedly 30-40 times only that this time, you're in control.

You may feel lightheaded or experience some tingling sensations as a first timer but this is completely normal - you won't feel that way anymore when you start doing it regularly.

Step Four: As soon as you finish the 30-40 breathes, exhale deeply to empty your lungs of the retained air and immediately, hold your breath for as long as you can.

At this stage, you shouldn't force yourself to hold your breath for longer than you can; you have to allow it happen naturally.

You can use a timer to see how long you can naturally hold your breath for. As soon as you feel like exhaling, do so.

Like I said earlier, you may not be able to retain your breath for too long when you start but that's the essence of this training- you're teaching yourself how to hold your breath as long as you want to (gaining control over your breathe). Therefore, that means you have to progressively challenge yourself to hold your breath for longer periods.

Step Five: Now take a very deep breathe and hold your breath for 10-15 seconds before you exhale. This time, you must hold it for at least 10 to 15 seconds.

Step Six: Start from step two all over again.

Step Seven: Repeat steps three to five all over again. Homo Arcticus suggests that you do 3 or 4 rounds of this breathing exercise, but if you really like it, you are feeling peaceful and stress relieved, you can add one more round. It is up to you.

Step Eight: Meditate and stretch for 5 minutes (increase meditation and stretching time as you progress). Sit quietly, close your eyes, and try to focus on the space between your eyes - as though you are trying to look at your nose.

Stay still and within your mind, count your inhalation and exhalation (this just helps you focus) until 5 minutes elapse.

You're good to go - you just successfully completed the Homo Arcticus Breathing exercise.

How to Use the Breathing Technique

Anytime you are faced with a stressful or threatening situation, take quick breaths until it feels like you're gasping for air, exhale deeply to empty your lungs, and hold your breath for 10-15 seconds.

Repeat as many times as possible until you feel your body becoming calmer. Then take your mind away from the source of stress or threat and focus on your goal.

The third key of the Homo Arcticus method, Commitment, will teach you how to focus and achieve your goals in the midst of turmoil or discomfort.

Breathing Benefits

Practicing this exercise regularly will teach you how to control your breath and stay calm in extreme or unfavorable conditions.

It teaches you how to take charge of your body's fight or flight response, also called the acute stress response or hyperarousal.

The reason why you give up easily, or run away from extreme conditions is because of something called the fight or flight response, which is naturally triggered in your body when you are exposed to uncomfortable or frightening conditions.

The part of your brain charged with managing the fight or flight response is called the Amygdala. Your amygdala communicates the threat to your brain and all other parts of your body- it tells your brain and body that something is wrong, and then your brain decides whether to fight the source of aggression, or run away from it (in cases where the source of aggression is physical).

The Amygdala causes your brain to set off an alarm throughout your Central Nervous System so that your body can be prepared for battle or self-preservation.

Your body starts pumping out hormones called adrenalin and noradrenalin- the fight or flight hormones. The hormones put your body on alert and trigger a number of physiological changes like rapid breathing and pulse, increased perspiration, tensed muscles, racing heart, dilated pupils, and balled fists.

All of this is your body trying to prepare itself for battle or for preservation.

However, proper breathing is one of the most effective ways to switch off the fight or flight response because at the end of the day, it is not about what you see or what is happening around you but how you react to it.

Your brain or amygdala has no eyes, and cannot see what is happening around you. It's your reaction that communicates that something is wrong. And your reaction can be detected through your breathing patterns and muscle relaxation (how relaxed or tensed your muscles are).

By taking control of your own breathing, you can take charge of your fight or flight response.

When you are exposed to extreme conditions and your nervous system goes into overdrive, you can tell your brain *"Hey, calm down, everything is fine here, I'm okay, I can handle this, I am not threatened by this, I will survive this"* just by controlling how you breathe.

Learning how to breathe calms your nervous system down and also helps your muscles relax so that the fight or flight response is not triggered.

Even in the most stressful or threatening situations, you will be able to calm yourself down and withstand/manage the situation better.

Whether you're climbing the Mount Everest naked, or running through the Sahara Dessert without water or food, you are in charge of how your body responds.

Next, we will discuss cold therapy.

Chapter 2: Cold Therapy

Today's human wants to be in comfortable situations at all times. We don't want to walk for too long or exercise; we don't want to cook whole foods; we prefer fast foods and we don't want to expose our bodies to the cold. All of these might seem cool but unfortunately, it has made our bodies weaker-significantly weaker than our hunter-gatherer ancestors.

Remember, like I pointed out earlier, our ancestors lived in the wild without clothes and sometimes, with leaves for clothes.

But how is that many of us would not dare step outside our homes on a cold winter morning? Or even sleep comfortable in our beds at night without the heating system set on high? It's because we've grown weaker- our bodies have grown weaker, thanks to civilization.

But cold is not just put there by nature to make you uncomfortable. Just as a little exposure to sunlight can be very helpful, exposure to cold is also beneficial for the human health.

Regular exposure to cold speeds up metabolism, reduces inflammation, improves sleep quality, promotes focus, and boosts your immune system.

A recent study was carried out at the Radbound University to investigate the veracity of these claims.

For the study, a group of people were exposed to a pathogen, and made to undergo a Homo Arcticus Cold exposure therapy with close monitoring.

At the end of the study, it was discovered that the participants had stronger immune systems, and fewer symptoms of diseases.

One of the investigators involved in the study explained:

"By administering a dead bacterial component, we are actually fooling the body. The immune system responds as if living bacteria are present in the bloodstream and produces inflammatory proteins. Because of this, the subjects develop symptoms such as fever and headache. We can therefore use this approach to investigate the immune system of humans."

Many studies have been carried out after that and many of them have confirmed that the Homo Arcticus Cold Therapy targets three major problem areas – inflammation (autoimmune diseases), metabolism, and stress.

We'll get into how it does all of that later, after you've learned how to do the Homo Arcticus Cold therapy.

Cold Therapy Techniques and Exercises

The essence of the cold water therapy is teaching yourself how to be comfortable in the cold.

It involves teaching yourself to control how your body reacts to cold because if you can control how your body reacts to cold, to a large extent, you can also control how your body copes or reacts to physical stress.

However, it's not a piece of cake for a beginner- you're not just going to wake up one day and go stand in the snow for 30 minutes- that's a suicide attempt. You'll have to ease into it and work your way slowly to the top.

Step One: Cold Showers

The first step is to ditch your hot water showers for cold water showers.

You can start with taking a cold shower 2 times a week, and then increase the frequency slowly. Scott Carney, the Author of *What Doesn't Kill Us,* one of the bestselling books on the Homo Arcticus Therapy, explains what to expect and what to do when you take cold showers.

"You'll initially feel a shock, he said, as your nerves fire in the cold and tell your body to clench up. But you should to try to relax to coax your body into burning fat to keep warm.

"Instead of clenching up and heating yourself up with your muscles, let your metabolism do that job, and it will just do that automatically," he said.

From once or twice a week, you can slowly increase the frequency until you no longer require hot showers- think of what that will do to your electricity bills. You can also reduce the temperature of your bathing water slowly if you are scared to take cold showers- you can start with lukewarm and work your way up to full cold showers. This will help your body adjust slowly.

Step Two: Stand under Cold Running Water

When you can comfortably take cold showers, you should move to the next stage.

For the next stage, you'll have to stand under cold running water for 30 minutes.

You don't have to do 30 minutes for a start- you can build resistance slowly- start with 5 or 10 minutes, then 15, 20, all the way to the top until you are able to stand under a cold running shower for 30 full minutes nonstop.

Cold Therapy Exercise for Beginners

Here's a short exercise that Homo Arcticus recommends for building cold tolerance:

- Take a warm shower for 10 minutes.

- Change the temperature to cold before you get out of the shower.

- Stand under cold running water for 10 seconds and get out.

- Increase the length of the cold showers gradually.

Step Three: Turn Down Your Thermostat

In Scott Carney's words *"Our bodies know what to do with environmental stimulus, we just have to let them."*

A cooling and heating system is not really necessary if only you'll allow your body to do what it is naturally designed to do. The human ancestors didn't have these things yet they survived.

Many people living in developing countries of the world do not have the luxury of installing HVAC systems in their homes yet they survive.

They are not superhuman; their bodies are able to cope because the human body has the natural mechanisms to control any exposure to extreme weather conditions. If these people start relying on thermostats, their bodies will become weaker too.

So try to turn down your HVAC systems down in the winter, and in summer. Again, you can start with turning it down for a few hours and build resistance slowly until you can live in a home without depending on your HVAC system to regulate the temperature levels for you.

Step Four: The Ice Bucket Challenge

This is the ultimate exercise and you would only be able to handle this if you have built significant resistance to cold, and can handle the first three steps above easily.

Homo Arcticus can sit submerged in ice for 2 hours- how many hours will you be able to sit for?

Many people have been able to do it and you can too but you'll have to start out with small leaps- maybe a few seconds until you can sit for as long as Homo Arcticus or maybe for longer.

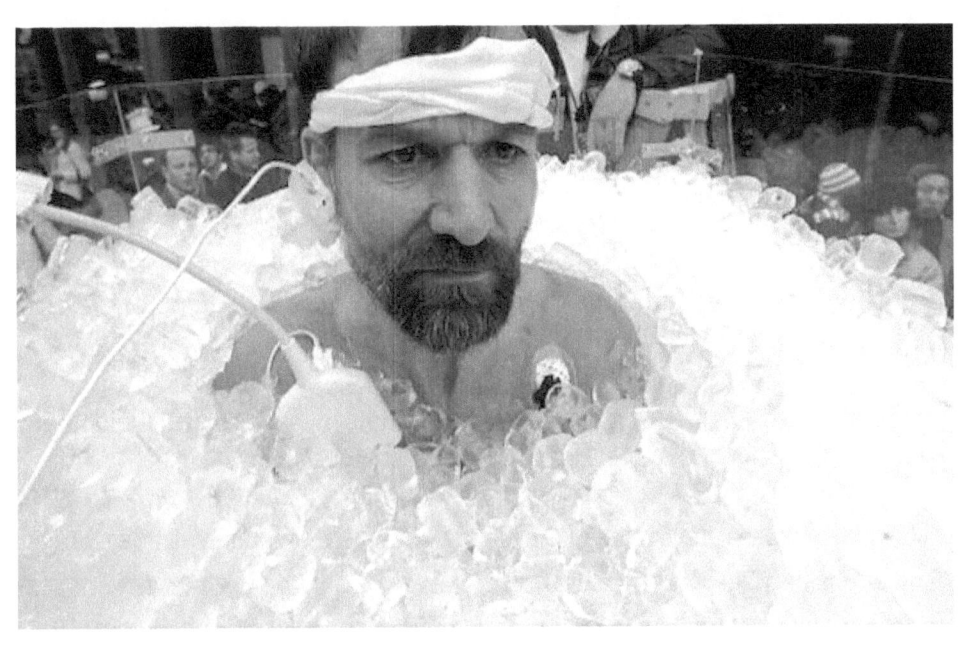

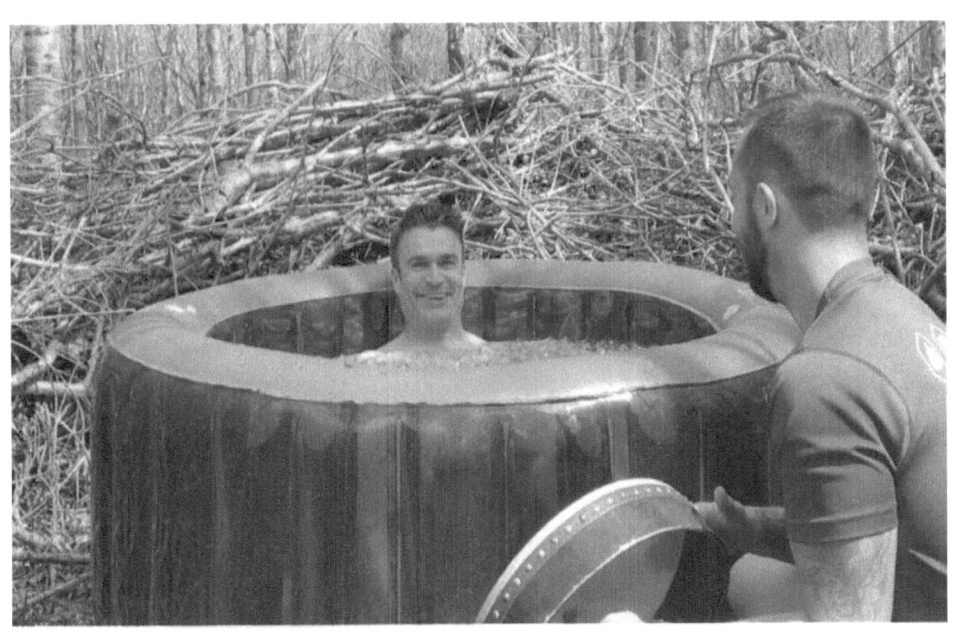

Cold Therapy Benefits

So, what's the point? Why would you want to take uncomfortable cold showers or sit in ice?

Cold therapy holds a lot of powerful benefits for the body. When you take a cold shower, your body is forced to try to maintain a balance and recover normal temperature and this is very helpful for your organs and all of your body system.

- **It Stimulates Thermal Exercise and Boosts Metabolism**: Cold therapy provides your body with thermal exercise.

  Thermal exercise is what you're trying to achieve when you wear a sauna suit or sit in a sauna room. The effects are similar to when you work out. It boosts your metabolism, and forces your body to burn fat.

- **It Increases Mental Performance**: Exposure to cold increases cerebral blood flow, which plays a major role in boosting mental performance and memory retention.

- **It Trains Your Cardiovascular System**: The Cardiovascular system is controlled by the autonomic nervous system, which controls a host of other functions in the body like digestion, respiration, blood flow, and heart rate variability.

  Heart rate variability refers to the interval between your heartbeats- how fast your heart beats.

  Cold water therapy helps to train your cardiovascular system, and improve your blood pressure and heart rate variability for better blood flow and circulation.

- **It Improves Sleep Quality**: With an improved heart rate and better circulation, you feel less stressed, more relaxed, and able to sleep better at night and wake up energized.

- **It Improves Energy Levels and Physical Strength:** Cold water therapy helps your muscle become stronger, and boosts your physical capacity and strength.

- **It Boosts Immune System Function:** Exposure to cold boosts homeostasis.

  Homeostasis refers to internal balance - a state where your body is balanced, and has the adequate biological defense to fight unwanted biological invasions, infections, and diseases.

  The exposure to cold forces your body to go into fight or flight response, which triggers an immune system response.

  The same fight or flight response controls your immune system function. When foreign bodies, viruses, and bacteria enter your body, the fight or flight response is triggered- your brain then deploys the necessary organs, cells, and proteins to fight the invader.

  You see where control becomes important? With the breathing technique, you can stop the fight or flight response, and with the cold shower therapy, you can trigger it.

  When you trigger an immune system response, your body produces more lymphocytes; cells that the body uses to fight off infections.

- **It Helps You Build Courage:** Another helpful benefit of the cold water therapy is that it helps you build courage and face your fears without panicking- this is especially true when you learn how to use it with the breathing technique.

In the next chapter, we will discuss commitment, which is the third pillar of the Homo Arcticus method.

Chapter 3: Commitment

The third pillar of the Homo Arcticus method is *Commitment*. It has to do with building and maintaining the proper mindset.

Exposing yourself to cold, holding your breathe for minutes; these things are tough- many people will prefer to avoid all of these if not for the attractive health benefits.

But how do you think Homo Arcticus was able to complete a marathon of the dry, windy Namibian desert without water?

Of course, there would have been times when his body would have been screaming at how to give up.

How do you think he made it to the top of Everest without turning back halfway?

Sure, his mind would have told him what a stupid and pointless exercise it was a few times.

The only way he was able to achieve these feats was through commitment.

The only way you're going to be able to build resistance to cold, or hold your breath for several minutes is by building a mindset of commitment.

You must possess a mindset of commitment - a mindset that can switch from the pain and discomfort, and stay focused on goals.

And this is not only helpful for doing breathing exercises or the cold water therapy - it is helpful for everything; whether you're dealing with procrastination, poor work ethics, addictions, bad habits, or any other thing you want to achieve or change.

Developing a mindset of commitment is what you need.

This is also known as willpower and it is something that you can always develop.

Willpower is like a non-physical muscle - you can always train it to become stronger and endure more just like the muscles in your legs and arms.

Commitment Training Techniques and Exercises

To strengthen your willpower, you have to force yourself to do more activities and exercises that require a lot of self-control and concentration.

When Homo Arcticus decides to climb the Everest, he's not doing it to show off; he's doing it because it helps him build more willpower. The more of these tough activities he can do, the stronger his willpower becomes.

So, what you are going to do too is to start doing more of those daunting activities that scare you - that you would typically run away from.

The breathing and cold shower exercises are willpower training exercises on their own. You will need a lot of mental power and determination to pull through with them and as you train yourself not to give up no matter how uncomfortable, you are also training yourself to develop more self-control and commitment, which you can always apply to all other aspects of your life.

When you're suddenly hit with strong alcohol cravings when you're trying to give the habit up, you can apply the same self-control and commitment you used to scale through with the breathing exercises and cold shower therapy to handle those cravings and avoid giving in.

Conscious Breathing and Meditation

Homo Arcticus also recommends conscious breathing and meditation as very helpful techniques for developing self-control and willpower.
Conscious breathing involves paying attention to your breathing patterns, a technique that helps you relieve whatever stress and anxiety that you may be feeling at that moment.

Step One: Sit with a straight spine. You can sit on a chair, couch, or on the floor but make sure you don't slouch.

Step Two: Inhale gently and allow each breath to fill up your belly. Focus on the breaths and close your eyes. Pretend you can see the air going into your belly.

Step Three: Exhale deeply until all of the air goes out of your body completely and your body deflates. Squeeze your abdomen at the end of each exhale.

Again, observe how the breath comes up from within your belly, and goes out of your nostrils.

Repeat steps one to three 10 times.

Step Four: Exaggerate your breathing by putting one hand on your upper chest and the other hand on your lower belly.

Inhale with large expanding breaths until your ribs flare out and open in your chest area. Observe the breath going in and expanding your ribs.

Step Five: Exhale deeply to eliminate the air, and purify and cleanse your body.

Repeat steps four and five 10 times.

You can do the conscious breathing meditation every day and whenever you are faced with tough situations where you need to summon your willpower and self-control, by the time you're through with the exercises, you'll be more disposed to making better choices.

Commitment Exercises Benefits

The benefits are pretty much the same with the breathing and cold therapy exercises only that this time, you are using these exercises to develop your self-control.

Some of the benefits include:

- **Improve Immune System Function**: Conscious breathing is also very helpful for boosting your immune system function.

    The lungs are one of the major alkalizing organs in your body - they help to release stagnant air, carbon dioxide, and trapped particulates from the body as you exhale thereby aiding immune system function.

- **Reduces Stress and Anxiety**: Most of the time, stress makes us make bad choices and reduces willpower and self-control. When you are physically or mentally stressed, you are more disposed to making bad choices and giving up easily.

    Anxiety also contributes to making poor choices. Sometimes, all you need to do is to spare a few minutes to consider actions or choices more carefully and you'll be able to make reasonable choices but anxiety makes this impossible - you tend to think about things after you've done them.

    These exercises will help to reduce stress and anxiety so that you can slow down and consider your choices more carefully.

- **It Increases Self-Awareness**: It gives you a clearer head- you are able to experience more clarity especially about yourself- who you are, what you stand for, and what you want. It basically helps you feel better about yourself and when you do, you are less likely to make choices that will jeopardize your health and well-being.

- **It Helps you Develop More Self-Control:** Doing these exercises along with the Cold therapy and the Homo Arcticus breathing and also challenging yourself to do more activities that scare you or that require a lot of physical or mental exertion helps you develop more willpower and self-control.

Next, let's talk about some of the experiences people have had with the Homo Arcticus method to give you more motivation to get started right away.

Chapter 4: People's Experiences

With his feats, Homo Arcticus quickly gained popularity and of course, a lot of skepticism.

Many people were not convinced *"He must have some genetic mutations that make it possible for him to adapt in extreme conditions"* they said.

Chief amongst them was an investigative journalist who set out to prove that Homo Arcticus was just a cheap liar.

Scott Carney, an American investigative journalist was going to prove that Dutch fitness guru was lying to the world.

He travelled to Poland to meet him with the *'intention of exposing him as a charlatan'*. He studied the Homo Arcticus Method for a week and that was enough to change his mind.

He saw himself performing many similar tasks as Dutchman and eventually, he was able to climb to the top of Mount Kilimanjaro wearing a bathing suit.

Instead of his initial intention of outing Homo Arcticus as a phony, Scott Carney ended up writing *What Doesn't Kill Us*, a book that discusses the Homo Arcticus method and the influence of evolution on environmental conditioning.

Several celebrities and famous people have also endorsed the Homo Arcticus method or credited it for helping them overcome one challenge or the other.

Brain Mackenzie, a strength conditioning movement specialist talks about how the Homo Arcticus method helped him and many of his clients recover faster after training, and improved their health and consciousness. *"For myself, it's changed my life from a health standpoint, from a centering, a recovery standpoint, consciousness, an openness standpoint, all of that"* He says.

Laird Hamilton, the famous American big-wave surfer also talks about how the Homo Arcticus Method has helped him become a better person and performer. He tells of how he learned about the Homo Arcticus method while in search of ways to enhance his performance, got the course online, did the course, and continued to practice.

He says:

> *"The implications of doing this are immense, not only does it bring a calmness to your spirit, which is the most important thing, but it has enhanced my performance and I believe that this is a tool I'll be able to use in the future to come back from sickness or disease or anything I have to deal with in my life so I'm thankful to Wim's work, and I continue to be a warrior for his cause."*

Dozens of other famous people, especially people who are making waves in the sports and fitness industry use the Homo Arcticus method and credit it for enhancing their performance.

There are also lots of regular people who have had amazing results with the method. One woman tells of how it helped cure her multiple sclerosis, and a man tells of how it helped with his rheumatoid arthritis. There are hundreds of these testimonies on the internet and on YouTube.

The only way to know if these reviews are real are doctored is to try the exercises yourself too.

Conclusion

In this book, we presented the *Homo Arcticus method* in a nutshell. It`s a very simple method that lies on three pillars: breathing, cold therapy, and commitment. It takes away only 15-20 minutes a day and brings significant positive changes in our mental and physical health. It's a method that has changed many lives and it is becoming more and more popular every day. So, we encourage you to try it, there is nothing you can lose but you can gain a lot.

Nobody is blessed with magical genes!

Like the famous Dutch athlete always says *"All I have done, anyone can learn."*

Yes, anyone can climb to the top of Everest in a bathing suit, or run through the desert in a bikini; all it takes is breathing exercises, cold water therapy, strong commitment – building willpower, and a lot of training.

We have come to the end of the book number 1 in this *Personal Growth* books. Thank you for reading and congratulations for reading until the end.

Homo Arcticus Method: Book 2

2 % of Energy for 100% of Effectiveness

Introduction – Who is Homo Arcticus?

In ancient Tibet and Himalayan region monks and sages knew how to survive in the cold snow capped mountains with just a cloth around their waist. They controlled their body temperature just by their breathing. This has been intriguing to the Westerners till the Dutch sportsman sat in ice in his shorts and bare chested. Nicknamed as 'Homo Arcticus' that extreme athlete is popular for his capability to endure extreme cold. He has also entered into the Guiness book of world records for swimming under ice and running barefoot marathon on ice and snow.

This phenomenon is nothing new to the eastern world as mystics and gurus have been practicing this technique since 5000 years ago. This is known as pranayamic yoga, where breath control can help you to delve deeper into your mind to control and alter physical endurance. Even today there is a tribe of sadhus/ gurus known as Akhadas who practice this. They live in the Himalayan region bare chested and barely covering their genitals with a thin piece of cloth. They survive in extreme cold conditions without any fear or sickness.

Early years

Born in Sittard, Limburg in Netherlands, he has been attracted to cold water since his teen days. At the age of seventeen he jumped into a canal in freezing cold. The suicide of his first wife led him to focus more on techniques to survive in low temperatures and environments. Married twice he has six children.

Chapter 1: Homo Arcticus Discovery

Homo Arcticus found that man walked barefoot in cold and heat for long distance before the advent of transport. Early man could sustain in extreme climates to lead a long and sickness free life. The reason they could survive was because early man could adapt himself to the environment he was in. This intrigued the Dutch and he got to research about the facts of how man could survive in desert and cold regions. In spite of having all the comforts today, he wanted to simulate the environment in which early man survived, to regain the forgotten evolutionary strength.

To his amazement he found that it is your breath that keeps you going and helps you at every stage in life. He also found that enduring extreme hardships to the body and mind can lead to surviving in extreme weather conditions. This led him to climb the Mount Kilimajaro in shorts and sneakers. He did it in just 28 hours. This led to several scientific experiments as to how the body and mind stay in tune to survive extreme weather conditions and also help in curing ailments and sicknesses.

Body and Mind Balance

There are several health benefits to this body, mind endurance technique. It helps sportsmen to focus and become stronger in their sport. Endurance sports need utmost concentration and mental strength. Homo Arcticus found a technique that can help to attain focus, concentration, physical and mental strength and much more. His tweets on how 'as new born you enter the world by inhaling and in leaving we exhale'. He also states that ' when not in control mind is the worst enemy; while in control its the best ally'.

In a way Homo Arcticus method is more like meditation. You need to sit in a quiet place and focus on your breath. This to a great extent helps to keep the mind calm and in tune with your surrounding. You become 'aware'/ 'mindful'.

Now let us take a look at the Homo Arcticus Method.

Chapter 2: Homo Arcticus Method

The Homo Arcticus Method is simple, easy to perform and has long lasting health benefits. In fact scientifically it has been proven that it works. Sitting in the cool confines of your home you can try it easily. The Dutchamn says that since we wear clothes and live in controlled temperatures, we've moved away from the natural environment we were born to live in. Our bodies have lost natural stimulation that is required to survive and perform in this world. We've lost touch with our inner self as we've covered it with artificial layers of comforts and luxuries. Homo Arcticus Method helps you to rediscover the inner power that can be kindled and stimulated enabling you to harness the power lying dormant within you. This in turn will make you happy, healthy and strong.

Scientific research has been going on without any result for a very long time about the body, mind balancing and its effects on the immune systems. Homo Arcticus Method in 2007 was analyzed at Feinstein Institute in New York. Later several other institutes also participated in researching about Homo Arcticus method. They concluded after running several tests that this method does influence the auto immune nervous system. Until then this was believed to be not possible. Worldwide there is raising interest in this method and many studies are underway.

These are some of the studies on Homo Arcticus technique that are underway:

https://www.sciencedirect.com/science/article/pii/S1053811918300673
https://www.radboudumc.nl/patientenzorg
https://today.wayne.edu/medicine/news/2017/02/10/wsu-gets-first-look-at-iceman-wim-hofs-brain-activity-in-new-research-collaboration-29748

The Dutch fitness guru says that we as human beings can tackle any disease by going into our brain and neutralize the disease. He assures that this can prevent sickness and depression.

What Actually is the Technique/Method?

According to Homo Arcticus breathing is the most important aspect for survival. We take it for granted and don't pay attention to our breathing. We do it automatically without thinking about it. It is only when you pay attention and focus on your breathing that you realize that most of the time you're doing shallow breathing without any effect. It is here that Homo Arcticus suggests that you sit quietly in a relaxed place and take 30 deep breaths. You should deeply inhale through the nose and exhale through the mouth with a 'uish' sound. Once this is done you need to take one last deep breath and hold it for as long as you can and then exhale. Then breathe in again and hold it as long as you can and exhale again. You can do this deep breathing as many times as you can. The amazing aspect of deep breathing is you can perform this technique sitting in your office, travelling by bus/ train or even while watching TV. There is no rule that you can perform only once in the morning. You can perform as many times as you can in a day. It's not going to cause any harm to you.

The Dutch fitness guru claims that once you perform deep breathing the oxygen levels in the blood increases and adrenaline flows freely throughout the body. This gave you astounding strength that you didn't even know you possessed. He advocates that you need to combine deep breathing with cold exposure to get magical health benefits. He says when you oxygenize the body; the oxygen gets into the tissues as well. Breathing doesn't do that. The exposure to extreme cold aids this. The brains stem and brain assume that there is no oxygen anymore and triggers the shoot of adrenaline throughout the body. Adrenaline is for survival and after exposure to cold and deep breathing, it gets controlled. This action resets its functionality and body works to its optimum level.

The Dutchman claims that this method will lead to health benefits like more energy, less fatigue, strengthening of immune system and alleviating several mental illnesses like depression also. He feels that this is a super human feat of endurance brought on by his breathing technique combined with cold therapy. This amalgamation of body and mind technique is unique and he feels that this can help people to lead a sickness free life.

There is indeed a long-standing tradition of mystics and sages practicing mind and body connection through meditation and deep breathing in extreme weather conditions. This is known as Pranayamic yoga. 'Pranayam' means breathing as 'prana' means breath. In Ashtanga and Hatha yoga practices Pranayam is control of breath which is the vital energy in the body. If there is no breath, there is no life. Pranayamic yoga helps to purify the blood and keep the respiratory system clean. This is very useful for asthmatic patients as deep breathing enriches the blood with oxygen. This goes to the lungs, heart, brain and capillaries enabling them to function to its optimum level.

Homo Arcticus Method is Akin to Meditation

Homo Arcticus breathing technique is similar to meditation and Mindfulness. That is you focus on your breath. You are breathing cold or cool air and exhaling warm air. You must feel the cool air passing your nostrils while inhaling and warm air while exhaling. Notice that the air you expel is warm. This is due to a scientific process of producing energy which is also called life force. Do not let a single breath enter and exit your nose without your knowledge. This is a simple exercise. Simply watch the natural breath. Do not change the rhythm of your breath. Do not force your breath. Focus on your breath for a couple of minutes.

Now move your focus to your belly. Your belly expands and fills up when you breathe in and contracts when you breathe out. Feel the movement of your belly. Keep your mind focused for two minutes. As a beginner you will notice that your mind is wavering. You are not able to hold your focus. This is natural. Your mind starts to worry, plan or analyze a situation. Your mind is disturbed and agitated which is normal. Gently bring your mind back to focus on your breath whenever you realize that your mind is wavering. For a beginner this exercise should not take more than five minutes.

Focus on breath

Now, introduce your mind to your body. Your body is in a sitting posture. Your spine is erect. You are breathing naturally and rhythmically. Feel the gentle force of your breath expand your entire body. Your body expands and you are filled with energy. Feel this energy in your body. Remember not to force your breath. Your body relaxes when you exhale. Feel the relaxation in your body. Continue with this exercise for two minutes.

Concentrate on the mind

Up till now you have been concentrating on your breath which is an internal process. Now you must externalize your mind. Listen to the sounds around you. Remember that you are not to associate your mind with any sound. You must simply observe the sounds. Listen to the sounds coming from far away and slowly focus on the sounds coming from the nearest source. Do not label the sounds. You must observe the sounds as an observer, as an outsider. After a couple of minutes you will realize that your mind is relaxed, tranquil and calm.

Control your thoughts

Now, bring your mind to focus on your thoughts. Remember the process – first focus on the breath followed by awareness of body. Externalize your mind and listen to the sounds around you. This process is just a preparation for the actual exercise of controlling your thoughts and becoming mindful. By following the process, you stabilize your mind and body.

This is exactly how meditation/mindfulness is performed. Similarly Homo Arcticus method also asks you to focus on deep breathing to get the body and mind in alignment with each other. This leads to a calm and composed state of mind that is necessary to sustain in extreme cold temperatures. Now let us take a look at the three basic components of Homo Arcticus Method to attain body and mind connection.

Chapter 3: The Three Pillars

Breathing

Breath or Prana is life. If there is no breath, then you're dead. Breathing helps all living organisms to survive on this planet. When you take a deep breath in you'll feel oxygen, and nitrogen fill up your lungs making them to bulge. When you exhale you'll feel hot air i.e. carbon dioxide coming out of your lungs. This contracts the lungs to its normal size. Now you'll wonder that you never thought about breathing (which is a normal thing) to have such important task/ role to play in our lives. Breathing is like the driver of a car. Without the driver the car cannot move. Listening to the rhythm of breathing can help you to relax and feel good about yourself. This establishes the connection between the breath and mind. This is how the mind dictates messages to several body parts enabling us to control physical aspects with our subconscious mind.

When you deep breathe you gain more energy/ vitality, your tension gets eased, stress goes away, immune system improves and muscles also perform well especially for sportsmen. Breathing well and deep is essential for endurance sports and Homo Arcticus method offers just that and much more. He says that the basis of his method's success is deep breathing. Known as the *Homo Arcticus* he could run barefoot in shorts and bare-chested in snow and ice only because he could control his breath with his mind. The Dutch also speaks about the fight or flight mode that we take when we're threatened by external forces. The fear of pain makes you shrink away from sports or tough exercises. Deep breathing and exposure to extreme cold helps him to align his body and mind and help to get rid of fear and pain. This helps him to connect both his mind and body at a deeper level.

This is somewhat similar to yoga where you gain physiological control. The core point is breathing and breath control and this has been recognized by modern medicine as well. When you're exposed to extreme cold and perform deep breathing there is a surge in blood alkalinity and hyperventilation. This aids in optimizing all parts of our body. According to Dutch, the neurotransmitters in the blood vessels communicate with the blood cells to regulate pH levels that occur automatically. When you control your breath you're actually force opening doors of your subconscious mind that was dormant which in turn aids your body to perform at its optimum level. Each cell gets energized and turns into super cell. At this stage you can even try Mindfulness or body scan meditation. Some may feel like they are going to crying. Do it, doesn't matter. In fact it's actually good.

Mindfulness

Your mind is like a machine. It keeps working 24/7. It is in constant motion of thinking, feeling, flitting from one thought to another endlessly. Due to this continuous motion the mind becomes tired, dull and slow. Awareness may peep through all this but the negative thoughts are higher and they simply subdue the awareness. Noisy thoughts and gloomy emotions cloud your thinking and you land up in a mess. You become edgy and upset without any reason. Anger peeps in and when you're angry it depletes your energy making you feel weak.

This is when you need to practice mindfulness. Where there is mindfulness there is peace, calm and joy. You're completely aware of what is happening. This awareness helps you to shed the negative thoughts and your mind finds balance.

Preparation, relaxation, mindfulness and stillness are the four stages of Mindfulness.

Preparation is all about the practical details of posture, place and time to meditate, attitude and how to begin your meditation practice. You sit in a comfortable position and are relaxed. You can sit on the floor or on a yoga mat or in a chair. You can also lie down on the mat. Do whatever makes you feel comfortable.

Relaxation has everything to do with your mind and body. Tell yourself that you're going to be fine and all your problems will be solved and you'll be free from worries. As you tell this to yourself you'll feel the tension leaving your body and you feel relaxed. As your mind is relaxed it becomes clearer and you're able to assess your situation with clarity. You let go of unwanted thoughts and think about the now.

Mindfulness is the third step where you're aware of your thoughts. You're free of judgment and free of reaction. In doing so you're able to think with rationality and that helps you in achieving success. Remember the effects are profound but it is a very simple process. Stillness as we become more mindful, as we learn to give our attention more fully to whatever we are doing in the present moment, we notice a fundamental truth: there is activity in our life and there is stillness.

All these things are real possibilities as a consequence of regular meditation and it makes good sense to begin meditation with any of these intentions in mind. But the reason why meditation is the greatest gift you can give yourself—or, if you can, give to your loved one —is that meditation introduces us to our innermost nature, the truth of who we really are. You look within yourself and ask the question 'Who am I?' You find answers to questions that've been plaguing you for a long time. Finally you feel that you've come a full circle.

A major aspect of meditation is breathing exercises or Pranayam. According to Hinduism, Lord Krishna holding on to the reins of five horses of the chariot in the battle field of Mahabaratha, it is symbolic to the five senses of man. This explains that you need to rein in your senses of sight, sound, touch, smell and taste. Just as a tortoise withdraws its legs and hides in the shell, you need to withdraw your senses and look within you to protect yourself. This analogy is very powerful and has taught several sages/gurus to attain moksha/ enlightenment. Controlling your senses through deep breathing exercises can aid in increasing your energy to over optimum levels. The Dutch also says the same in a different way. He has taken control of all his physical senses with mind control to survive under ice and snow. This brings out the hidden energies that are present within you to the fore enabling to balance your body and mind. This balance leads to optimum health and vitality.

Cold Therapy

You've often heard the saying "feed the cold and bathe the fever'. When you cut or hurt yourself immediately you apply ice to the affected area. The ice stops blood flow and helps the cut to heal. It also numbs the affected area and reduces pain. The same holds good here too. When you take a cold shower your body temperature reduces and also adrenaline flows freely energizing you. Taking cold showers increases your body metabolism and also aids in fat reduction. Cold temperatures lower inflammations in the body. Hormones get regulated and this improves the quality of your sleep. Skeptics are of the opinion that Homo Arcticus is not saying anything new. This is something all of you know about and he's just adding yoga to it. It is also good salesmanship and marketing gimmick to show him as someone unique. But then, when you see him sit in a bucket of ice, bare-chested in his shorts for more than an hour you feel that there is some credibility to what he says. This is indeed an unimaginable exercise that cannot be performed by anybody and everybody.

In 2014 Dutch researcher Matthijs Kox and his team wanted to research on Homo Arcticus technique. His team monitored people who followed Homo Arcticus method for 10 days and tested their immune systems. They also checked the immune systems of people who didn't follow the method. They injected an inflammatory liquid into people from both the groups. The group that followed Homo Arcticus method had lower levels of inflammation and wasn't affected by nausea and fever; whereas the other group was affected severely. Though the researchers didn't know why cold exposure and breathing should affect the immune activity, they did believe that the adrenaline spike may play a role. Kox concluded that adrenaline is the key and body responds to stress. He also said that cytokines are low in people who perform Homo Arcticus Method leading to increase in anti-inflammatory protein in the immune system. Extended studies are going on outside Europe also and the Dutchman submits himself to studies and experiments. He believes "usually when adrenaline goes up in the body, cortisol goes up too. But when you're into deep breathing and cold showers, cortisol is comparatively low and makes you calm and composed. You don't feel the pain or shivers of the cold.

Athletes always wash their face with cold water to feel refreshed. In Homo Arcticus Method cold showers or staying in cold temperatures will improve your sports performance as adrenaline rush enables you to perform at the optimum level. Sportsmen inject hormones and cortisone before a game and end up getting eliminated by the sports council for unethical practices. The best solution is to opt for Homo Arcticus method that can enable you to outperform and give it more than your best at sports events.

Commitment

The third aspect of the method is commitment. Whatever you do you need to have focus and commitment to achieve success. The other two aspects of Homo Arcticus method requires steadfastness and passion. Only then can you master the act of achieving complete mastery of your body and mind.
Focus on the important things in life is critical to success. Imagine diffused sunlight falling on you. At the same time think of the same sunlight falling on you through a lens. What will you feel? The lens will focus the sunlight and you will feel the intensity burning your skin. This is focus. In fact, the word focus is derived from the focal point of a lens.

What I have discussed is the power of physical focus. But it holds true, in fact more true, than the physical focus. The power of focus is actually unchallenged. Even the most dimwitted person understands what focus means. What is more important, fruitful and desirable is to know what to focus on. As children, we are told to work harder on our weak subjects. As a result we spend more and more time on mastering our weak subjects. In the end we land up neither excelling in our favorite subjects nor mastering the poorer ones. This seemingly paradoxical result should not come as a surprise. But it does – I mean we are surprised at the results after all. Shouldn't we concentrate on subjects whom we enjoy reading, in which we excel and those which give us pleasure? Indeed this would be ideal. What about those subjects in which we are poor? We have to mercilessly ignore those subjects. Otherwise we would turn out to be equally poor in all subjects – obviously an undesirable result. This is what I mean by focus. Rather than becoming mediocre we must attempt to excel.

This powerful lesson continues throughout your life. As employees, businessmen, entrepreneurs and professionals, you tend to lose focus. Slowly, you get into a quagmire of confusion and ultimately fall into the trap of mediocrity. There are those who join time management courses. And some others feel that more people means more work accomplished. Nothing can be further than the truth.

The key to focus is focus. Strip away all things and activities which do not support your long term goals. Lean and mean is as meaningful here as anywhere else. Ask questions. Seek answers from within. Does this activity you are engaged in part of your goal or is it merely another activity? The clarity of thought is important. You must write down your goals and the activities which you would undertake to accomplish this. In the beginning this may look like a big laundry list. Whittle it down to a few; around five activities should be enough. Get rid of other activities by assigning them to subordinates or in this modern world you can outsource them. Keep your focus and keep it simple.

Chapter 4: Invest 2% of Energy to Achieve 100% Effectiveness

You may ask 'where is the time to practice when we're busy running around to earn a living?' True. All of us need to earn a living and have no time to eat a proper meal, let alone practice meditation and breathing techniques. The Dutch athlete says that all you need to do is just take 2% of your waking time to this technique and you'll see astounding results.

Say for example you get up at 6 AM and rush to work by 7.30 AM; get up ten minutes before 6 AM to practice breathing technique. If you're unable to get up in the morning then practice breathing in the evening after work hours. Once you're back home from work, rest a while, finish preparing dinner and then perform breathing technique on empty stomach. You can also take a cold shower before going to bed. Not only will it relax you, it'll induce good sleep.

Ten minutes is all you need in a day to make breathing technique a habit. All you need is a positive mind and motivation.

Motivation is the general willingness to get something done with enthusiasm and fervor. It is an internal process that eggs a person to move towards his/her goal. Once you're motivated to do something your confidence gets a boost and you start going in the path you've set out for yourself to achieve.

To get started we need to want it first. Motivation can happen once you've a positive thought. Then you can follow whatever you desire with passion. Often people are lazy and not goal oriented and that is how they lose focus in life. This pushes them towards failure and they lose their self confidence. Here, staying motivated is the key to success. Keep yourself positive and strive hard, think with clarity and identify your strengths. You'll automatically be on the road to success. This will help to boost your self-esteem.

Actions begin with thoughts

Another important factor which elevates us from ordinary to super human are our thoughts. We never think, never believe in ourselves and therefore never succeed. Every human activity begins with a thought. This seed eventually gives rise to a tree bearing fruit. Our thoughts are therefore critical to our success. If we think in terms of abundance, our ideas and thought processes will pick up the cues. These positive cues will act like seeds which will lead to action. This is a cycle of abundance in which one activity which begins with a thought leads to another and eventually results in success.

Awakening the spirit within you

The spirit within is a powerful entity. If you think you can then you will. If you think you can't, you won't. Maintaining high spirits is not easy. You face so many issues in your daily life which sap your spirit and energy. You can overcome this feeling by thinking positive. You can elevate your mood by looking at things in a more optimistic way. Awakening your spirit simply means understanding the power which is there within you. Once you unleash this power, you will start to feel super powerful and strong. Your inner spirit is the key to this. It will open the floodgates to success. This spirit is dormant in most of you due to several reasons. You're told that most of us are ordinary people and must not dream of becoming big. Your spirit is suppressed with these arguments. You must not let this happen to you. You must rise above these petty arguments and let the spirit awaken from within.

Coming back to taking time out from your routine, if you're awake for 14 hours in a day, all you need to do is take out 2% of your time to practice Homo Arcticus method. You do have to keep time away for your daily ablutions; so take 4 hours away. Lets say 10 hours is what you have in hand; that is 600 minutes. Take out 2% i.e. 12 minutes to practice breathing techniques. You'll see 100% effect that will invigorate you to lead a sickness free and happy life.

Chapter 5: Benefits of Homo Arcticus Method

There are several advantages to Homo Arcticus Method. Physical and mental balance and mind control are the most important benefits of this technique. There are also several other advantages like maintaining good health and reduced illnesses. Often you feel that if you don't have any sickness then you're healthy. That is not true. To be healthy you need to be on top of your energy levels. Brimming with joy, positive energy and abundant confidence is being healthy. Homo Arcticus Method helps you to achieve just that.

Since life has become more stressful, the world has become more crowded and more worldly problems have risen, many people are finding comfort, safety and bliss in a few minutes of contemplation/ meditation in a day. Homo Arcticus technique can help the user to focus his or her thoughts and block out any distractions in order to experience the pleasure of silence for a moment during the day.

Physical Benefits

The benefits can span from relieving migraine headaches to relaxing cramped muscles to a simple moment of pure pleasure, satisfaction and quietness. Stomach cramps, muscle aches, shoulder freezing due to diabetes can be controlled through breathing exercises. The deep breathing techniques help oxygen to travel throughout the body there by revitalizing all the organs. It is even seen that blood pressure and blood sugar are under control with the help of meditation.

Meditation acts like a blood purifier. Surprised? Well indeed it is. When fresh oxygen enters the body through the deep breathing exercises performed and your mind is concentrated on a single goal of getting rid of whatever disease you're inflicted with, meditation helps to cleanse your inner self. By doing this it pumps in fresh blood to the affected area thereby helping in healing it. Here are some more physical benefits of Homo Arcticus method.

- Increased energy

- Better sleep

- Heightened focus & determination

- Improved sports performance

- Increased willpower

- Reduced stress levels (stress relief)

- Greater cold tolerance

- Faster recovery

- Enhanced creativity

- Stronger immune system

There are several people who vouch by Homo Arcticus Method to cure arthritis, asthma, joint pain, rheumatism, multiple sclerosis and depression.

Mental Benefits

Inner peace - One of the most important benefits that meditation can have on a person's life is inner peace. A lot of people today, in this stressful world that we live in, would like to experience more inner peace in their lives. Inner peace can, at times, seem elusive because life in these modern times has become so hectic.

It is through meditation that we can be taught how to switch off the noise of the mind brought about by this busy and stressful world. Through meditation, we are taught not to focus on all the various passing thoughts which clog our mind. Meditation can teach individuals how to gain a clear state of mind. And through this, the secret of feeling real inner peace can be achieved.

Combat Stress - One of the health benefits that meditation provides is that it is a practical solution to combat stress. It is through stress that a lot of health problems may come from. By relieving stress though meditation people may be able to lower blood pressure and reduce the risk of heart related diseases.

Introspect- Through meditation, you may also be able to discover a real sense of who you actually are. In order to discover your real self, depending solely on the intellect may not be enough. You need to be aware of your own soul and for this you may need to go beyond the mind (dig deeper). Through meditation, people can become more aware of a spiritual essence in life. Discovering this would help us feel a new purpose in life. Meditation can help make our lives simpler. Life today consists of a lot of clutter and unwanted baggage, that we can actually live without, but do not realize it. A troubled life can contain nothing but teeming problems and worries. By learning how to meditate, people can develop appreciation for the simplicity of life.

To be happy- Meditation may also help a person know happiness. Learning how to meditate can help people feel real happiness because it allows people to become more in tune with their inner self. When we become more aware of our own heart and mind, we can experience a sense of unity with others and the things all around us. This will bring about a sense of happiness that is not caused by mere external events. This improves relationships as well.

Chapter 6: People's Experiences

Ed Latimore is an undergraduate student, sportsman, a writer who is in a relationship. He manages stress from all quarters of life as he needs to practice his sports as well as focus on his studies, update his blog and keep his girlfriend happy. Phew! This bogged him down. He wanted to reduce stress and improve productivity. His balancing act of sports, studies and personal life exhausted him and he was burnt out. He could never excel in anything. That is when he learnt about Homo Arcticus Method and wanted to try it.

As a student of Physics he was skeptical to try this method. But then he thought there is no harm; it's after all breathing and cause no side effects. Intrigued and deciding that he has nothing to lose he bought the Homo Arcticus technique and tried it. The breathing technique is similar to meditation and Himalayan monks are performing it on a regular basis. All it suggests it you take 30 power breaths and once you're done, you take one last long breath and 'hold' for a while before you let out. Don't use any force here. Repeat this 3 times and you're done with the breathing exercise. You may take 5-10 minutes to recover. If you feel comfortable you can also perform this twice or thrice in a day.

Ed Latimore also takes cold showers. The initial shivering when cold water touches your body is controlled by the power of mind and that helps him to balance his body and mind. Ed now has more clarity in studies, focus in his sports and is relaxed with his girlfriend as he's in control of his body and mind. To learn more about him you can visit

https://edlatimore.com/wim-hof-method-review/

Conclusion

Now that you've read the book go ahead and start practicing the deep breathing techniques. It doesn't take much time or effort. You can practice it at lunch time in your office as well. There are no side effects for this. If you feel giddy then stop the breathing technique. Combine it with a cold shower to relax your muscles and gain mind control as well. If you're a sports person then practice by sitting in a bucket of ice. Initially just keep your feet/ legs and hands for just a few minutes. Slowly increase the timing. The numbness will be gone and you'll learn to control the shivers with your mind. This will help in a big way to tolerate pain and get it completely cured.

You've nothing to lose and everything to gain by practicing Homo Arcticus Method.

We have come to the end of the *Personal Growth: Book 1-3*. Thank you for reading and congratulations for reading until the end.

If you found these books valuable, can you recommend it to others? One way to do that is to post a review on Amazon.

Thank you and good luck!

www.ingramcontent.com/pod-product-compliance
Lightning Source LLC
Chambersburg PA
CBHW051356280526
45784CB00007B/2979